HOW I TO
& YOU CAN, TOO!

STEALING
your
healing

SHIRLEY ANN WEIDENHAMER

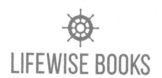

STEALING YOUR *healing*
How I Took Back My Healing & You Can, Too!
BY SHIRLEY ANN WEIDENHAMER

Copyright © Shirley Ann Weidenhamer 2019. All rights reserved. Except for brief quotations for review purposes, no part of this book may be reproduced in any form without prior written permission from the author.

Published by:
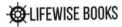
LIFEWISE BOOKS
PO BOX 1072
Pinehurst, TX 77362
LifeWiseBooks.com

Cover Design and Interior Layout | Yvonne Parks | PearCreative.ca

To contact the author | www.windowsofheaven.info

ISBN (Print): 978-1-947279-65-0
ISBN (Ebook): 978-1-947279-66-7

dedication

To God be the glory:
Jehovah Rapha,
the Lord who heals.

To my husband, Ray:
The best husband I could ever hope for,
the man of my dreams.

To my children:
Todd, Jeffrey, Kristin, and Matthew,
I love you.

acknowledgments

I want to thank my wonderful husband, Ray, whose endless love and support for me was always there in every way. He did the endless cooking and delicious soup making—thank you. I love you forever.

My special friend and secretary Dana Hood, who volunteered her help in any way I needed and volunteered her heart of encouragement so often through this process. Thank you from the bottom of my heart.

Thank you to my daughter Kristin, who renovated and designed "Shirley's She Shack," as she named my writing room, and surprised me with it one day. Thank you to Phil, our son in law, who helped immensely with his computer skills as well as renovation of the writing room.

And to my special friends, Dan and Mary Evans, thank you for your support and belief in me. You warmed my heart and life.

table of contents

Introduction	9
Chapter One | Someone Stole My Health	11
Chapter Two | Avenues of Healing	27
Chapter Three | Declare War	43
Chapter Four | Move Those Mountains	57
Chapter Five | Wow, God, Wow	67
Chapter Six | I Dare You	83
Chapter Seven | The Beginning of the Beginning	95
Conclusion	107
About the Author	111
Endnotes	113
Works Cited	119

INTRODUCTION

Like the woman who touched the border of Jesus' garment in Luke 8:44 and stole her healing, I chose to do the same. This is the story of how I stole my healing back. I admit it is not easy, but it is doable. *Stealing Your Healing* is a journey you might want to take also. You can take it—yes, take it back. For the woman who has the passion and the commitment to overcome the fear of dreaded disease, or any other heartbreak, I write this book.

I was diagnosed with breast cancer. Perhaps, you may have experienced another case of stolen goods, like your finances, your relationships, your sanity, your peace, your joy, or your hope. I learned these can be taken back. Cancer is a word that strikes fear in the heart of a soul, the fear of death. I received my healing one step at a time by going to God for the strength and the peace His Word brings. Daily, I repeated out loud the scripture which says, *"[I am] strong in the Lord and in the power of His might,"* [1] and *"by whose stripes [I was] healed."* [2] I declared this truth as my daily, hourly, and even minute-by-minute statement of faith. I spoke to this mountain of disease called cancer and told it to, "Die at the root, and get out of my body." It had to obey me—it had to go. No matter what I feel, no matter what the facts are, truth wins.

The Word of God is a real, living Word that heals. It is as real for today as it was back then. God's words are real to everyone who believes. Like the woman with the issue of blood, we may *"declare unto Him before all the people for what cause we have touched Him,"* that He will say unto us, *"Daughter, be of good comfort: thy faith hath made thee whole: go in peace."* God cannot lie. I invite you to follow along with me on this journey of learning how I took back my health, through the practice of God's Word.

chapter 1
SOMEONE STOLE MY HEALTH

I WANT IT BACK

I was sitting on a gurney in the doctor's office, chatting with my daughter. The door opened. Without a greeting, the chilling words of the doctor broke the atmosphere of pleasantry. Ringing in my ears were these words, "You have breast cancer, and you need an operation." His next words were, "Choose either a mastectomy or lumpectomy with radiation." He further announced, "We need to do it this week, or next week." With my heart racing what felt like a hundred beats a minute, I could not hear what he said after that. I could hardly take a breath. Someone had stolen my health.

Has your health been stolen? The truths I found for taking my healing back are for anyone. I feel the intense desire to share with you the steps I took to take my life, my health back.

Fear of that dreaded word, "cancer," was all over me. I was frightened. "How can I fight through the fear? How can I overcome it? God, help me," was my first response. "I need your help, God."

He reminded me of the record in Luke 8:43-48 about the woman who touched the border of Jesus' garment and took her healing. I love this record; it has been an inspiration to my heart and life. The account reads:

> *"And a woman having an issue of blood twelve years, which had spent all her living upon physicians, neither could be healed of any, came behind Him and touched the border of His garment: and immediately her issue of blood stanched. And Jesus said, 'Who touched me?' When all denied, Peter and they that were with Him said, 'Master, the multitude throng thee and press thee, and sayest thou, "Who touched me?"' And Jesus said, 'Somebody hath touched me, for I perceive that virtue is gone out of me.' And when the woman saw that she was not hid, she came trembling, and falling down before Him,*

> *she declared unto Him before all the people for what cause she had touched Him, and how she was healed immediately. And He said unto her, 'Daughter, be of good comfort: thy faith hath made thee whole; go in peace.'"*

This woman took her healing. She showed great courage because she was unclean and by law could have been stoned for even being in the crowd. I love her boldness. Imagine, she was under the threat of death, yet she went to the Master as her source of her healing. She was totally convinced that healing was hers. She took her healing when she touched the border of His garment. Jesus said that He "perceived that virtue," (power), went out of Him. Her faith had made her whole.

Cancer patients have that same threat of death spoken over them with every diagnosis. Instead of fighting for their life, which is a common plan, I propose a paradigm shift: know that healing is yours biblically and take it back; therefore, "stealing your healing." Receive what is rightfully yours. If the Word of God offers healing, then you can legally take it; it is a gift of God.

A friend gave me a pretty present wrapped nicely for my birthday. When she handed it to me, I simply accepted it. It was a gift. I didn't have to do anything special to earn it or deserve it. I did not have to beg, plead, hope, or pay for it, I simply and thankfully took it.

Healing is a gift from our precious heavenly Father and His Son, Jesus. *"By His stripes ye were healed."* [1] Unwrap and enjoy God's gift to you; it is yours

HOW DO I GET IT BACK?

My husband and I make our decisions together. I fully admit this one was a huge challenge. How would we handle this mountain? After much prayer and discussion, we decided we would take God at His Word. He cannot lie. His Word is true, and He is faithful to His Word. We put our faith in total agreement with Him and His Word.

Acting on that Word was what lay ahead. Fear was the worst thing. How was I going to resist the fear? With God's direction, my husband and I laid out our journey. I wanted to believe I received my healing immediately when I prayed. I didn't want to pray and then endure the excruciating wait for the doctors' reports. Now was the time to become fully persuaded with no doubt, no fear, no worry that words in the Bible would now be a living, life-giving, healing reality. My health had been stolen from me. I had a passion to take it back. My prayer is that my journey will help any of you who desire to take your health back also.

Every day my husband and I would pray together. For fifteen minutes each day, we visualized my taking the steps of victory, like a champion in a movie. I declared, "I have the victory." We both spoke in tongues while picturing the victory of a clean bill of health. We found a verse, a living Word of God, in Romans 4:17b that says we are to *"calleth those things which be not as though they were."*

"I am healed," were the words we spoke to that mountain of disease. We did this daily for a very long time. We did go to God with every step we took before we acted. My doctor gave me a choice. After going to our Father God, we decided on the lumpectomy with radiation. I know that not every case is the same, and other choices may be given, but I was trusting that after going to God for my direction, He would direct my steps.

"Thou will keep Him in perfect peace whose mind is stayed on thee, because he trusteth in thee." [2] We chose to believe and receive His peace, which helps calm any fear of the future. So, I began acting on that Word. I know I must have called on that peace thousands of times along my journey. It was not easy; no, it was not. It was doable, however, and I refused to be frozen in fear. The lion had roared, and I knew that if he could freeze me in his tracks, he had me. But I stayed with the Word of God.

Now, I refuse the fear when it comes, and it does come. It also goes for a time. I learned to submit to God and resist the devil, and he had to flee. If he doesn't leave, we have not resisted. However, my enemy of cancer did flee. Thirteen years later, I can confidently handle the fear that tries to jump me. He has tried many times, but I have submitted to God every time. The devil has fled, just as God's Word promises.

Since I am a veteran of the United States Air Force, I was in their care for the surgery and radiation. The nearest veterans' facility was almost two hours from my home town. I had to stay in a motel for six weeks to receive the treatment five days a week. Being away from my loved ones was a huge challenge. My family all worked, and I do not drive.

However, I was never alone. My faithful and awesome God never left me. He showed how well He could handle these difficulties if I would simply put my trust in Him.

God provided friends during my stay who would take me to my appointments, out to a restaurant, or dinner in their homes. Several people volunteered to take me shopping, and some even took me on sightseeing tours of their town, to the movies, and to Bible fellowships. One woman cleaned my motel room for me, making it nice and comfortable to live in. I received amazing love and care from so many wonderful friends.

There were many moment-by-moment choices for me to make in the face of fear and confusion. Was I going to elevate my circumstances and symptoms above the Word of God? Or, was I going to elevate the Word of God over my circumstances and symptoms? It was a fight, but a good fight of faith, to believe that I was healed.

SOMEONE STOLE MY HEALTH

IS HEALING MINE TO TAKE?

Now I do not believe in stealing, but if healing is rightfully mine, then I know I have the right to take it back. I found a verse in the Bible that clearly tells me it is mine. I Peter 2:24 tells us Jesus paid the price. *"His own self bare our sins in His own body on the tree, that we, being dead to sins, should live unto righteousness: by whose stripes I was healed."*

Healing is mine. I am fully persuaded. Jesus Christ paid for it. I am not the sick person pleading for my healing, I am the healed who is taking back what the devil has stolen from me—my health.

We can all choose how we want to live since we have free will. Faced with cancer, I chose the Bible as my only rule of faith and practice. With His Word in my heart, my journey to prove healing is mine began.

I like parties, and I enjoy all the goodies on the food tables. Usually, I go for the dainties which I rarely have time to prepare—the specialty items, like the delicious pies and cakes. I love chocolate cake, but I rarely bake anymore. So, I go for that yummy, delicious, chocolate-frosted, gooey, chocolate cake above all the other beauties.

God has prepared a table for us with the delicious dainties of His Word. He has already prepared the feast, so all we need do is select what we want and take it. What did I want?

My selection was my vibrant health back, (my chocolate cake). Now, it didn't walk over to me on its own. I had to pray for my vibrant health or chocolate cake. Yet, I had to do one thing more, and that was to take what I desperately wanted. I had to take the first step, the second, the third. I had to take action or that gleaming, delicious, vibrant health (or chocolate cake) would not manifest in my life or in my mouth.

Believing is acting on the Word. When I take a big bite of that delicious chocolate cake, I am full of joy. Nothing else beats the flavor that so comforts me.

Psalm 23:5a says, *"Thou preparest a table before me in the presence of mine enemies."*

Reading these powerful words gave me the opportunity to take of His feast, my chocolate cake, my vibrant health. Oh, how sweet it was and still is—His Word to me. I think there is no greater wealth than my vibrant health—sweet like my favorite cake.

My poor health was from the enemy. With each delicious morsel of His Word, I could laugh louder at my defeated foe. He couldn't rob me of my blessings of health and recovery. I chose to partake from the feast, the table God prepared, savoring my vibrant health with great joy and thanksgiving.

What do you want to receive from God's table? His bountiful provision is available to you right now. Just take it. Receive it.

I always thank my host and hostess at a feast. I am so thankful for all they prepared that I could or would not fix for myself. Likewise, I thank my God for the feast of His Word spread out before me to freely take. It is all ready, and we are invited to the table. We do not have to pray a thousand prayers, do a thousand good deeds, or give a thousand dollars to receive healing. No! He already provided it. Just reach out and take it.

Remember the first taste of that specialty item you desire? While you savor the taste, you might say, "Yum, it is so good!" What praise you would have for the baker, your host or hostess!

What praise we should freely offer to our God who daily prepares and offers an awesome feast of His Word for us! We will never be able to thank Him enough. We were created to glorify Him. Oh, how He loves it, because He loves us so very much. He says, "Take and eat, my dear children; that glorifies me."

Here are more of His dainties, His healing words: *"He sent His word, and healed them, and delivered them from their destructions."*[3] *"Beloved, I wish above all things that thou mayest prosper and be in health, even as thy soul prospereth."*[4] God's will includes our health and prosperity in all areas of life.

We no longer need to say, "if it be thy will." His Word clearly says healing is His will. Why, then, are we praying, "If it be your will, please heal me"? That is a prayer of unbelief, which is contrary to His Word. He already gave His Word, and He does not lie.

The church is waiting for God to answer prayers for healing when He has already provided healing. They may think their prayers were not answered and say things like, 'It must not have been God's will." That answer places the responsibility of our believing on Him. No—we believe, we receive. Are we calling God a liar? He already told us His will. Why would we ask God to do what He has already done? Believing is what pleases Him. I decided I was taking my healing. I believed, and I received.

I found many verses which say healing is ours and it is His will. Find His healing promises in His Word, learn them, and live them. The healing scriptures we know are how many we get to take for ourselves. I have found many and have many more to go. The Bible is full of promises just waiting to be discovered. There are so many amazing truths we can search out and then apply. We can live in health, as it says in Proverbs 4:20-23:

> *"My son, attend to my words; incline thine ear unto my sayings. Let them not depart from thine eyes; keep them in the midst of thine heart. For they are life unto those that find them, and health to all their flesh. Keep thy heart with all diligence; for out of it are the issues of life."*

According to His Word, we can clearly see God's will is life and health. Our responsibility is to keep His Word hidden in our hearts just as we would hide a priceless treasure. His Words are life and health to all our flesh. Our life springs forth from what we keep in our heart. The heart is the innermost part of our being, where our believing originates. What a treasure He has provided to us! Life and health are rightfully ours. On my healing journey, I learned it is God's will for me to have health, and God has already made provision for me to take it back and keep it forever.

THE DEVIL DID IT

Who stole my healing from me? The thief was at work, and I found him. *"The thief cometh not, but for to steal, and to kill, and destroy: I am come that they might have life, and that they might have it more abundantly."* [5] Who is the thief? The Bible says it is the devil. *"Be sober, be vigilant; because your adversary the devil, as a roaring lion, walketh about, seeking whom he may devour."* [6] Your adversary, the devil, is the thief. Notice, he is seeking whom he may devour. He cannot devour us if we resist his methods. We resist *"lest Satan should get an advantage of us: for we are not ignorant of his devices."* [7]

His purpose is to steal, to kill, and to destroy. The devil stole my healing. His first intent was to steal, then to kill and destroy. He cannot kill or destroy if I do not allow him to steal the Truth of the Word of God from my life. I found the thief who did it. I uncovered his disguise and lies. Then the question became, how do I take it back?

What devices was I ignorant of? How do I resist the devil? These questions prompted my search. I needed answers. The adversary is a liar, the father of lies. My diagnosis was a fact. I did not deny the facts—I had breast cancer—but my prognosis was not the doctor's words, but rather the Word of God promising healing. By the truth of God's Word, now was the time to believe. Either I received my healing at the moment of my request, or I allowed the adversary to steal it away from me.

Truth trumps fact. The devil's plan was not just to make me sick—he planned to steal my healing, to kill and to destroy me. My plan was to find out how to defeat the works of the adversary on this journey and to steal my healing back.

To take my health back, I had to appropriate it. What does that mean? It means to take something for one's own use. There is action to this. Something must be done. No sitting around waiting. Mark 11:23 and 24 explain what it means:

> "For verily I say unto you, that whosoever, [that's you and me], shall say unto this mountain, Be thou removed, and be thou cast into the sea; and shall not doubt in his heart, but shall believe that those things which he saith shall come to pass; he shall have whatsoever he saith."

Notice that it does not say anything about asking God to do it. It clearly says you or I must do it. Otherwise, we would be asking God to do something that He tells us to do. We must speak. The word, "say" is used three times, "say," "saith," and "saith." God is directing us to speak out loud to our mountain. Most people ask God to remove the mountain of sickness or any other barrier in their way. He clearly tells us we are to command it to be removed. We do it. The responsibility lies with us, the believer.

The verbs "be removed" and "be cast" are in the imperative mood form. The word imperative is from the Latin word, "*imperare*," meaning to command. The word, "empower," is a relative of this word.

Notice the scripture in Mark says, *"shall not doubt in his heart but shall believe that those things which he saith shall come to pass."* What does "doubt in your heart" mean? Mark clearly says, "shall not doubt." The heart is the innermost part of our being. Our core beliefs reside there. We may have doubt in our mind, but we can refuse to let it stay there.

We can change our mind and therefore change our heart. So then, by doubting (questioning) our doubts; we can conquer doubt, worry and fear, which all result in unbelief. How, you ask? By having trust, confidence, and faith in God's Word. This simply means believing as God instructs us. Meditating upon the Word, memorizing it, and acting on it builds my confidence, and trust. Therefore, I must not be wavering between two opinions. I agree with God.

WE ARE COMMANDERS

Refuse to slip back into the old "thinking" habits to hope, pray, and wait. Right now, command the disease or mountain to leave now. Use your God-given authority and confidence, and it must go. This is a new mindset or paradigm shift of thinking and doing. Since I already have won the battle, I am now speaking from a place of victory rather than seeking it. I am not commanding God to do anything, I am obeying God's instruction to speak with authority and command the disease to go and stay away.

> *"Therefore I say unto you, What things soever you desire, when you pray, believe that ye receive them, and ye shall have them."* [8]

When do you believe the answer to your prayer? At that moment when you pray, choose to believe you have received. Not later, but right then. I used to pray and wait to see if the prayer was answered. Now I see that if I believe I received when I prayed, it is mine. I now picture myself healed—which is an interesting change of belief. I no longer need to receive a good report from a physician because my healing is already finished by the work of Jesus Christ. My good report comes from the Word of God.

So, instead of asking God to take away my mountain or sickness, I now exercise my authority to command it to leave. The problem must go when I have no doubt. The Bible says in Mark, *"when ye pray believe that you receive them, and ye shall have them."* God uses the word, "shall" because it is an absolute, it is yours. I chose to make this paradigm shift of belief, and it really changed my life. We cannot be a victim and a victor at the same time.

> *"Now thanks be unto God, which always causeth us to triumph in Christ and maketh manifest the savour of His knowledge by us in every place."* [9]

Therefore, I am a victor, and God caused me to triumph in Christ. Daily, I choose to be a victor. I am coming from the victory, not towards it. The devil is a defeated foe. His only power is in what I allow and his lies which I entertain. I say, *"I am healed."* Also, I have a healing Word of God that I trust to be living Truth. I believe I received my healing the moment I prayed. Healing was mine. Healing is mine. I have it; I took it.

You can take it, too. Just reach out take hold of it. And hang on tightly!

chapter 2

AVENUES OF HEALING

Healing is here and it is available today for you and I. Healing was provided spiritually for *everyone* in the atonement. I searched all these avenues to discover a promise, a scripture I could accept, take, trust and live by each day. You may find more for yourself during your search or you could pick from these:

> "Who His own self bore our sins in His own body on the tree, that we, being dead to sins, should live unto righteousness: by whose stripes ye were healed." (1 Peter 2:24)

We see that healing was provided spiritually by the finished work of Jesus Christ through His broken body. Now you and I need to take it for our own use. We don't need to pray as if it has not happened yet, because it has happened and is available to all who believe. God cannot give us something He has already given us. I just need to appropriate it (take it for my own use.) Taking it is not claiming it and claiming it alone does not make it guaranteed. However, taking something that is already made available spiritually is guaranteed and can be taken for one's own use.

While I attended Bible school one year, I learned the difference between claiming and taking a promise. Johnny was in a Bible study class with me seated in the last row. The Pastor held up a ten-dollar bill and said, "I promise the first child who takes this bill may have It." You can imagine the children all saying, "I want it, I want it, I claim it."

Johnny thought, "How can I get to the front of the room to take it with all these other children ahead of me?" He ran as fast as he could, and, jumping onto the stage, he took the ten-dollar bill from the pastor's hand. No one else took it; they all wanted it and all claimed it, saying only, "It's mine, I want it." But they pursued no action to take it. Johnny took it. No one else got the ten-dollar bill.

That was how I learned to take the healing promises. Just claiming or wanting my healing went out the window. I just took them.

I also read about this in a book written by E. W. Kenyon titled *The Hidden Man*: "Claiming the promises is not faith. Faith already has it. 'Claiming' proves that one does not have it yet. It is unbelief attempting to act like faith."[1] Simply put, claiming is to call or cry out. There is no indication in the word "claim" that you believe you already have it and are acting like it.

"As long as one is trying to get it, faith has not yet acted. Faith says, 'Thank you, Father;' faith has it. Faith has arrived. Faith stops praying and begins to praise."[2] E. W. Kenyon continues, "Notice carefully, Doubt says. 'I claim the promises.' 'I am standing on the promises.' This is all the language of doubt. Unbelief quotes the Word, but does not act upon it. We call this Mental Assent."[3]

Claiming is not a guarantee. All things are possible to him who believes and takes the appropriate action. Using the Word in your daily life is the secret of faith.

THE WORD HEALS

> *"He sent His word, and healed them, and delivered them from their destructions."* [4]

I took every opportunity to feed myself the Word of God. It is a wonderful avenue of healing. The one requirement is believing or faith.

Scripture tell us: *"For verily I say unto you, that whosoever, [you are a whosoever], shall say unto this mountain...."* [5]

Does it say you are to pray to God to remove this mountain? No. The scripture says that you say unto the mountain, (a mountain can be financial, physical, or mental), *"Be thou removed, and be thou cast into the sea; and shall not doubt in his heart, but shall believe that those things which he saith shall come to pass"* [6] shall have whatsoever he said.

The promises of God are voice activated. Our job is to speak it! Speak unto the mountain. Nowhere in this verse does it say, pray that God will remove the mountain. We are waiting for God to do something that He has told us to do. It is impossible for God to lie, so He cannot do something He has already done. We need not ask for healing from God when He has already provided it. We receive it with thanksgiving. Healing is ours.

> *"Therefore, I say unto you, What things soever ye desire, when ye pray, believe that ye receive them, and ye shall have them."* [7]

When you pray, believe you receive them. At that moment of prayer, we believe we receive. Receive is the Greek word *lambano*, which means "to take." [8] Does it say you must wait until you see God's answer to your prayer? No. Believe you receive at the moment you pray. What a beautiful Word of God to believe!

AVENUES OF HEALING

The Word heals. Many scriptures throughout the Bible say God's Word quickens us. *Chayah* is the Hebrew word meaning *"to make alive"* and *"to cause to happen what His word says."*[9] His Word quickens, which is to make alive. God's Word revived and saved in that day. It can do the same for us today as well.

> *"My soul cleaveth unto the dust: quicken thou me according to thy word."* [10]

> *"Consider how I love thy precepts: quicken me, O Lord, according to thy loving kindness."* [11]

> *"Unless thy law had been my delights, I should then have perished in mine affliction."* [12]

God's Word saved the writer from perishing in his affliction. How many times has this living Word of God saved us in our afflictions or distress? It is good to remember those victories in our lives. Memory is a powerful thing. When times are hard, previous victories revive confidence, faith and hope.

God's Word is life. It is also health or medicine to all your flesh. Laughter is good medicine for your soul.

> *"A merry heart doeth good like a medicine."* [13]

> *"Wherefore lay apart all filthiness and superfluity of naughtiness, and receive with meekness the engrafted word, which is able to save your souls."* [14]

When God's Word is engrafted, it becomes part of you. The Word of God cannot be separated from you. When it takes root, (in your heart), it becomes greater than disease, and healing is the result.

This Word of God is a living Word. It is a living, giving Word of life and health:

> *"My son, attend to my words; incline thine ear unto my sayings. Let them not depart from thine eyes; keep them in the midst of thine heart. For they are life unto those that find them, and health to all their flesh."* [15] *"Keep thy heart with all diligence; for out of it are the issues of life.*[16]

A good question to yourself might be, "How do I spend my time?" Or, "What do I see and hear most of my day?" If the answer is television, newspapers, games, or social media, you might ask, "What is my focus?"

All these activities vie for your attention. What time is left for keeping your heart with all diligence? What time is left to attend to His Word? Purposefully check what is going into your heart, for out of your heart comes the issues of life—issues like your health and wealth.

I choose what comes out of my heart by controlling what I put in it. Am I sick? Am I lonely? Am I broke? Changing what I feed upon then changes my life. It is my choice.

Simply stated, the Word of God is healing. It affects my life and health.

You might say, "Okay, but if I am still not manifesting or showing healing, then what?" Well, there is another avenue available called communion.

COMMUNION HEALS

Communion is another source of healing we can appropriate or take. Communion is a memorial service to remind us we have a two-part redemption. When we eat the bread during the communion memorial, we are reminded of what Jesus Christ accomplished for us by His bodily suffering. It is not God's will for us to be sick. Perfect physical wholeness is available to us through what Jesus accomplished by His broken body. At that moment of time, we can receive wholeness and healing by believing we are free from all sickness and disease.

The sacrifice of the Passover lamb had two parts: (1) forgiveness, in which the lamb's blood redeemed the children of Israel from the destroyer; and, (2) healing, in which the lamb's broken body brought physical wholeness to all who ate of it. When the children of Israel left Egypt after eating the Passover lamb, everyone was in excellent health. Jesus Christ was God's response to man's need for forgiveness and healing. He was and is our Passover. The sacrifice of the Lamb brought spiritual and physical deliverance to all who ate of it. After eating the Passover lamb, the children of Israel left in excellent health.

> *"He brought them forth also with silver and gold: and there was not one feeble, [wavering or stumbling], person among their tribes." (Psalm 105:37)*

Jesus Christ bore our sins on the tree. He shed His blood for our forgiveness from sins, that is why we can *"live unto righteousness."*[17] Forgiveness and healing is God's will for us. He forgives all our sins so that we have spiritual wholeness and fellowship with Him. He also heals all our diseases. *"Who forgiveth all thine iniquities; [sins], who healeth all thy diseases."*[18]

> *"The cup of blessing which we bless, 'Is it not the communion, [fully sharing], of the blood of Christ?' 'The bread which we break, is it not the communion, [fully sharing] of the body of Christ?'"*[19] Also, *"or he that eateth and drinketh unworthily, eateth and drinketh damnation to himself, not discerning the Lord's body."*[20] Also, *"For this cause many are weak and sickly among you, and many sleep."*[21]

Many die early because they do not recognize the second part of God's provision in redemption. Our healing has been paid for. The church today may not really teach this second part of our redemption because many don't believe in it. We should come to the communion table with a pure heart and no condemnation, with a heart to remember and receive forgiveness and healing by the finished works of Jesus Christ. God looks upon the heart. I took and still take communion often.

THE HEALING MIRACLE OF THE NEW BIRTH

I reminded myself often that health was mine at the new birth. The greatest avenue of healing is the miracle of the new birth talked about in Romans 10:9: *"That if thou shalt confess with thy mouth the Lord Jesus, and shalt believe in thine heart that God hath raised Him from the dead, thou shalt be saved, [made whole]."*

If I am whole, I lack nothing, and this includes health. We were made whole at the new birth. What a miracle of miracles. *"For with the heart man believeth unto righteousness; and with the mouth confession is made unto salvation."* [22]

Through Jesus's sacrificial death, we were redeemed from what may be known as the curse of the law. *"Christ hath redeemed us from the curse of the law, being made a curse for us: for it is written, cursed is everyone that hangeth on a tree."* [23]

Sickness and disease are curses; curses that Jesus Christ paid for with his life for you and for me. Healing is for all. I think you may already know what it means to change lordships.

I am no longer the lord of my life. Jesus is my Lord now. I am a child of the most High God, and He gave me His Word which He magnified, but above all, He gave me His name. Every book in the Word of God has Jesus Christ as the subject. Each book of the Bible gives me direction on following His lordship. It lays a clear path to follow to walk in health.

PRAYER HEALS

Prayer is another wonderful avenue of healing that God provided, prayer in the understanding, and prayer in the spirit. *"Pray without ceasing."* [24] Living in the spirit of prayer, the Word says, *"In everything give thanks."* [25]

Think about what comes out of your mouth! Is it praise to God, and thankfulness for all He has provided? Or, is it mumbling and complaining about what you do not have? What you believe and speak not only affects your body, but your immune system as well. Your words become either a blessing or a curse to you. *"Death and life are in the power of the tongue."* [26] It is important to know who determines whether you receive death or life. You have the choice. Your words should be chosen carefully before you speak. Ask yourself, "Do my words minister life or death?"

"Because that, when they knew God, they glorified Him not as God, neither were thankful; but became vain in their

imaginations, and their foolish heart was darkened." [27] Some may say they know God, but do they glorify Him? Or, do they glorify men? Or even, glorify certain diseases above Him? Is cancer greater than God? The words you speak are vital to your health and well-being. There are some diseases that will never be cured unless people learn to speak the language of health that the body understands. God's Word is infused into you by giving voice to His Word with your own mouth, and this is the language of health to your body. Remember, the promises of God are voice-activated. Choose to glorify God and be thankful.

If we count our blessings and remember how much God has blessed us, our imaginations will not be in vain or empty. Our imaginations will be positive and brilliant, not negative which results in a foolish darkened heart. Remember, we are to guard our *"heart with all diligence, for out of it [come] the issues of life."* [28] This includes issues like our health and our wealth.

Healing and forgiveness go hand-in-hand: *"And the prayer of faith shall save the sick, and the Lord shall raise him up; and if he has committed sins, they shall be forgiven him."* [29] Pray in the spirit, which means you should speak in tongues. Any person who has the new birth may do this. Prayer was one aspect of God's Word that was particularly helpful for recovering my health.

Praying with the spirit, or speaking with tongues, will build you up spiritually according to I Corinthians 14:4. It provides a quickening (a making alive) of the mortal body. Speaking with tongues also will give you rest; a recess to recover and refresh. Speaking in tongues helps us pray to God His way, *"for we know not what we should pray for as we ought."* [30] The Apostle Paul thought it important enough to speak in tongues more than all the church at Corinth. Try it out for yourself and prepare to see the results! These are only a few of the benefits of speaking in tongues, and I need them.

Prayer in our native language, or "praying with understanding," is also communion with God. We have a connection higher than ourselves. Oh, what a joy it is to hang out with God in prayer. Could you have a better friend? Could you have a better time than being together with our magnificent Father? Can you imagine how blessed He is when you spend time with Him? Can you even imagine God feeling blessed with our fellowship? It is our opportunity to tell Him how much we love Him, how thankful we are, and to minister to Him. Can you comprehend that we can actually minister to our Father God?

God wanted fellowship with us, His children. He does not call us His adults, He calls us His children. How endearing, how intimate a relationship He desires to have with us. He wanted children who would freely love Him and tell Him so. He wanted children to connect with and share with throughout the day.

You know how nice it is to spend time together with someone you love. You may also know how you can hardly take your eyes off that person or leave his or her presence even for a short time. That is how God loves you. He really, really loves you. He is so blessed when we really, really love Him. To know Him is to love Him. When we spend time with Him in His Word, we get to know Him better and love Him more. God is spirit, and we can connect to and worship Him in spirit and in truth. When we spend time speaking in tongues or praying in our understanding with Him, we show our delight in being in His presence. Likewise, He delights in our presence. What a fellowship we can have, and what better way to spend our time?

It seems that a very large amount of the prayers offered to God are asking, begging, and pleading for things, especially when our backs are against the wall. This type of prayer to God is a vehicle to ask God for something, not about a relationship with Him.

What if we changed our conversation with Him to a personal, intimate relationship in which we confide in and love Him, telling Him of our love and thankfulness for all He has provided? We might then make our primary use of prayer to love and minister to Him. What about having an intimate fellowship with God, speaking to Him with our greetings like, "Good morning, God. Let's talk"? In His presence is fullness of joy. It doesn't get any better than that to me. If we walk in that kind of love with Him, He would shower us with more blessings than we could ask for or even think about.

> *"Now unto Him that is able to do exceeding abundantly above all we ask or think, according to the power that worketh in us, unto Him be glory."[31]*

What is working in us? We have God in Christ in us. We also have the Holy Spirit, the same power that raised Jesus Christ from the dead. That is awesome.

MINISTERING THE GIFTS OF HEALING

Many ministered to me. I also ministered the gifts to others. Ministering healing to others is another avenue God has provided for us to follow. Yes, some folks are adept at this, but all who are born-again and filled with the gift of the Holy Spirit can do it. Because we were commissioned by Jesus, we were also given His authority and the ability to reach out to others. But it is the doers of the Word who get the results, not the hearers only.

Let's obey His Word, lay hands on the sick and see them recover. Notice in Mark 16:15-18 that God does not say pray for the sick. He says, *"Lay hands on the sick."* *"Go ye into all the world and preach the gospel to every creature."* [32] *"They shall lay hands on the sick and they shall recover."* [33] We have the power and authority to do the works of Jesus. Healing is a vital function of those works.

When we impart gifts of healing, something goes out of us with that touch—virtue, which is the power of God. God has no hands but our hands. He works through our hands and our words. When we lay hands on the sick and speak life to another, the same power that raised Jesus Christ from the dead goes out of us. Release that power; not your power but the power of God. Ministering gifts of healing is one thing and prayer is another. We can pray throughout the day speaking in tongues to build ourselves up, so we are prepared to minister fully-charged to someone else needing God's touch.

I found that I can believe to live in the ways of these healing avenues and live as the healed, not the sick. Pleading, begging or asking for my healing is not necessary because I already have it. Knowing this, I am now coming from a place of victory instead of seeking the victory. These are a few avenues of healing I took or appropriated into my healing journey.

Certainly, there are more, such as anointing with oil, going to the elders of the church, and many I do not know as of this writing. God's Word is unfathomable. He has provided everything we need.

chapter 3
DECLARE WAR

FIGHT THE GOOD FIGHT OF FAITH

My journey has changed to one of being a victor rather than a victim. No longer am I fighting for my life, but to keep my faith or believing. Do we have to fight? Yes. The scripture instructs us to fight, but it is described as a good fight. *"Fight the good fight of faith, lay hold on eternal life, whereunto thou art also called, and hast professed a good profession before many witnesses."* [1] My journey took a new direction. I declared war.

2 Corinthians 10: 3-6 tells us:

> *"For though we walk in the flesh, we do not war after the flesh: (For the weapons of our warfare are not carnal, but mighty through God to the pulling down of strong holds;) Casting down imaginations, and every high thing that exalteth itself against the knowledge of God, and bringing into captivity every thought to the obedience of Christ: And having in a readiness to revenge all disobedience, when your obedience is fulfilled."*

It is not a fist fight, or a flesh fight. It is spiritual warfare. I firmly declared: "Now is the time to bring every thought that is against the knowledge of God into captivity to the obedience of Christ in my life!"

It is much easier to be entertained by television every evening than it is to put God's healing Word into my mind and heart which takes concerted study and effort. My life is at stake, and changing habits is a good fight of faith. Therefore, it is worth the effort to me. The good fight now is to keep my faith by bringing every thought captive to the obedience of Christ. I was in a battle of the mind: what God said versus what the doctor said, or what the world or the senses said — this is the fight. Sometimes we put up with sickness. I no longer tolerate it. I fight it like the plague.

Declare war against and cast down those imaginations that come to mind. One thought that should be cast down is that the big "C" is a death sentence. So many wonderful people have died in fear of the very name of cancer. There is no room for fear. None. You can't have faith and fear at the same time.

One fear that jumped on me was the fear that it could return. Even though the operation was successful, the fear of the big "C" returning kept coming to mind. The world says there is always the possibility that it might return. I chose the Word and resisted the imaginations that whispered, "what if it comes back?" The fight, the good fight was to keep my faith, my belief in His Word. I still often repeat what the Word says, "By His stripes I am healed."

Check every thought against the Word of God. Submit yourself to God and resist the devil. His lies must flee with him. The devil's one purpose is *"to steal, to kill, and to destroy."* [2] He wants to lower your resistance so that you give up the good fight. If you accept his lies and choose to accept the "C" diagnosis, you can lose your healing and possibly your life.

The doctor might say, "That is all that we can do; get your affairs in order." No, no, no. I heard the medical diagnosis and prognosis, but I did not, and I will not take them into my heart.

When I changed my focus, I also changed my life. I decided to take God at His Word. I was no longer pleading with God to heal me, but entertained new thoughts of thanksgiving to God for the healing He already provided. I stopped focusing on feelings and symptoms but rather on the truth of His Word. Some days I did not feel good, and some days I fought being frightened by a forthcoming test result. But I remembered each time, I was not fighting for my life, I was fighting for my faith—the good fight of faith (believing).

I am very thankful for my physicians and my nurses. They were very skilled and comforting. Because God is the source of all healing, my husband and I went to God on every step of the healing journey before we agreed to each procedure. There were only two procedures they offered which we went with another choice.

The truth is we are the healed taking back our healing, not the sick fighting to get healed. See the difference? With Jesus' crucifixion and resurrection, we already have the victory. Every one of my statements has a scripture truth to back it up. It is a choice to take and receive or reject His words of victory. I no longer plead or beg God to heal me—I praise Him for what He has already provided. The devil is a defeated foe. He cannot access us unless we allow him to by our open door of doubt, worry, and fear. Instead, I declare that, "I will have confidence, trust, and faith in the Word of God. It is impossible for God to lie."

The Bible says in Hebrews 6:18, *"That by two immutable things, in which it was impossible for God to lie, we might have a strong consolation, who have fled for refuge to lay hold upon the hope set before us."* I am going to fight the good fight and trust God's protection and His Word, while abiding in His refuge.

The devil can and will try every way he can to talk us out of our faith in God's promises. He is relentless, but he must flee when we resist. He may return, but we have the weapons of our warfare to use, to stand.

"I will fight the good fight of faith," is my declaration.

WEAPONS OF OUR WARFARE

> *"Finally, my brethren, be strong in the Lord, and in the power of His might. Put on the whole armour of God, that ye may be able to stand against the wiles of the devil. For we wrestle not against flesh and blood, but against … spiritual wickedness in high places. Wherefore take unto you the whole armour of God, that ye may be able to withstand in the evil day, and having done all, to stand. Stand therefore, having your loins girt about with truth, and having on the breastplate of righteousness; And your feet shod with the preparation of the gospel of peace; Above all, taking the shield of*

faith, wherewith ye shall be able to quench all the fiery dart of the wicked. And take the helmet of salvation, and sword of the Spirit, which is the word of God. Praying always with all prayer and supplication in the spirit, and watching thereunto with a perseverance and supplication for all saints. And for me, that utterance may be given unto me, that I may open my mouth boldly, to make known the mystery of the gospel." [3]

As children of Almighty God, we have weapons. We are equipped. We have the victory.

During my fight, I took every thought captive with my inner strength in obedience to Christ and put on my weapons of warfare to declare the victory in the face of the enemy. Was it easy? Sometimes, no. When the report from the doctor did not agree with the Word of God, no, it was not easy to manage the fear that came to freeze me in my tracks. Nor was it easy when the enemy perched on my shoulder and whispered in my ear, "See, all that declaring the Word of God does not work. You still have symptoms."

No, it was not easy, but it was doable. The simplicity of it was and is to stand, having on all the weapons of His warfare and do it all.

Personally, I am not moving off the Word of God. I am a doer of God's Word. I will not listen to or believe the enemy's lies. My God is faithful. I will stand permanently on His Word.

ROADBLOCKS

Unforgiveness

Shortly after my diagnosis, a dear friend invited me to attend a conference with her. There were many ministers and teachers there that I met for the first time. It was exciting, and I had high expectations for signs, miracles, and healings to occur. Ministering healing was an important part of the conference. I got ministered to, and to my surprise, the Minister had a word of knowledge. She explained that all kinds of fiery darts had been shot through me. Those fiery darts that had penetrated me represented hurtful words or deeds from people who had hurt me in the past. The darts had hit me at times when I did not have my shield of faith in place to protect myself. Those weapons had pierced through me causing destruction of my body.

I was encouraged to go home and write down the names of those people, including myself, who had hurt me in the past. Next, the minister said, "Forgive them. Forgive every one of them, including yourself if needed." She added, "Pray for and speak in tongues for each one of them daily for thirty days."

I obeyed her instructions and what a deliverance that was! I was free, free from condemnation, free from heavy burdens, and free to receive my healing with manifestation.

Unforgiveness is such a powerful barrier to receiving healing in any area of life. Once I exercised my right to forgive everyone, I was then able to receive. I began to speak words of life: "I believe I receive my healing." And I received.

What then, if you do not receive your healing? Then ask God, "What is the roadblock?" He will show you what has blocked your progress. He will guide you to what you need to do to gain your victory.

Fear

Fear is the worst roadblock to any freedom…physical, mental, spiritual or financial healing. A vivid illustration of this is in the book of Job. *"For the thing I greatly feared has come upon me, and that which I was afraid of is come unto me."*[4] The record begins,

> *"And there born unto him seven sons and three daughters. His substance also was seven thousand sheep, and three thousand camels, and five hundred yoke of oxen, and five hundred she asses, and a very great household; so that this man was the greatest of all the men of the east."*[5]

Job was a very prosperous man. He is described as *"perfect and upright"* and that he feared or respected God, and *"eschewed evil,"* [6] or shunned it. However, Job allowed fear to enter his life over his children's behavior of feasting and drinking. He began offering burnt offerings, and said, *"'It may be that my sons have sinned, and cursed God in their hearts.' Thus did Job continually."* [7]

Author James Allen wrote in his book *As a Man Thinketh*, "Thoughts of fear have been known to kill a man as speedily as a bullet, and they are continually killing thousands of people just as surely though less rapidly. The people who live in fear of disease are the ones who get it."[8]

We may have issues in life that tempt us to doubt, worry, and fear which result in unbelief. We then will have a roadblock to our healing. To clear out and conquer the roadblock, we must put our trust, confidence, and faith in our God and His Word. Fear can jump us any time; and we cannot allow it to remain. We can capture it and get it out. *"[Cast] all your care upon Him; for He careth for you."* [9]

Also notice that *"Thus did Job continually."* [10] Job's behavior gave the devil access to his life. Eventually, Job did become aware of and recognize that he had a roadblock. He said, *"'For the thing which I greatly feared is come upon me, and that which I was afraid of is come unto me.'"* When circumstances in life spring upon us bringing fear, we must cast our care and repeat Proverbs 3:5-6 to ourselves out loud:

> *"Trust in the Lord with all thine heart; and lean not unto thy own understanding. In all thy ways acknowledge Him, and He shall direct thy paths."*

Here is a real gem, *"I sought the Lord, and He heard me, and delivered me from all my fears."* [11] I began to fight my good fight by submitting myself to God and resisting the devil's roadblocks that I had not even thought of before. God opened my eyes to His Truth of protection.

RESIST THE DEVIL

> *"But He giveth more grace. Wherefore He saith, God resisteth the proud, but giveth grace unto the humble. Submit yourselves therefore to God. Resist the devil, and he will flee from you."* [11]

Once I realized what was happening, of course I wanted the devil to flee. I was so mad at him. I wanted to stomp on his head, however, I didn't know exactly what to do at that point. First, I fell helplessly at the foot of the Cross. I asked my Father for His divine help and submitted myself to resisting the enemy God's way.

> *"And when the tempter came to Him, he said, 'If thou be the Son of God, command that these stones*

> *be made bread.' But he, [Jesus], answered and said, 'It is written, Man shall not live by bread alone, but by every word that proceedeth out of the mouth of God.'"* [12]

Resisting requires humility to make the necessary adjustments in our thoughts and in our words to line up with the Word of God. God does not lie whereas the devil is the father of lies. I chose God's Word over the devil's lies.

The devil laughs as he says, "You're not going to make it."

God lovingly says, "You will triumph in Christ." I began resisting Satan with the Word of God.

I resisted the enemy in other ways also. I changed my diet to include healthy, fresh vegetables and fruits. I purchased organic foods as often as I could. I exercised at least 20 minutes every day. I cut sugar from my diet and developed an "I can do" attitude. With every step I took, I thanked God for everything I could think of or see. I started a journal to record my many blessings each day. I read His Word daily and maintained a close endearing relationship with Him. I was led to get plenty of sunshine outside and plenty of sunshine inward with lots of laughter.

I remember the story of Norman Cousins in his book titled *Anatomy of an Illness*. He had a life-threatening disease that medicine could not cure. His doctor said he knew of another medicine that could cure him, if he would do it. He then told him to memorize this scripture, *"A merry heart doeth good like a medicine:"* [13] He then told him to go to the library and get some old, classic comedy movies like Laurel and Hardy. While watching these classic comedies, he was to enjoy some good knee slapping laughter.

Afterwards, the doctor examined him and recorded the result of Norman's merry and joyful action. Norman was cured and became a living example of doing the living Word of God and getting positive results with his health.[14] That is some good medicine. I did the same. Indeed, laughter was good, and a merry heart was good like a medicine.

All these actions are ways to resist the devil who plans for us to feel sorry for ourselves, to be sad and depressed, with a "woe is me" attitude. We must choose to fight the good fight with an "I can do" attitude. People may think we are strange, but we can laugh at him anyway! Then, command the devil to go, in the name of Jesus Christ. Satan has endless suggestions that he throws at us—things like, "You aren't really healed, you still have pain. Nothing you do will heal you."

Say, "No" to the devil, "In the name of Jesus Christ go!" Then, speak the Word of God to him and to yourself. "I am healed."

I planted those words once and for all deep in my heart. The Word of God is truth, and the devil is a liar. To humble myself before God, I needed to adjust in my own healthcare. When I made these changes, I began seeing results immediately.

I learned the meaning of a quote from an anonymous source: "Pride makes excuses, and humility makes adjustments." I continued to do all that I could, following James 4:6: *"Submit yourselves therefore to God. Resist the devil, and he will flee from you."*

That's a promise. I took it. I believed it. I stood on it. Now, I share it with others who need a miracle.

chapter 4
MOVE THOSE MOUNTAINS

WHAT YOU SAY IS WHAT YOU GET

"Death and life are in the power of the tongue: and they that love it shall eat the fruit thereof." [1]

Spoken words have great power. Words hold the power of life and death. Because I am in control of what I say, I hold a powerful responsibility. Therefore, if I am going to have what I say, I had better pay attention to the words I speak.

My health was being stolen, and I was determined to take it back. I decided to begin saying what the Word of God said instead of what the world said. I did not declare the disease to be "my cancer" and I did not own it. Yes, the diagnosis was a fact, but the prognosis I believed was that I am healed. It is truth from the Word of God. Plain and simple, I believed I received no matter how I felt or what I saw. I began holding onto and meditating on the scripture in Romans: 4:17b, and to *"[call] those things which be not as though they were."*

Some of the most important things you speak are the words you say to yourself. Pay attention to what you are saying. There is no situation in which you are not able to triumph in Christ. *"Now thanks be unto God, which always causeth us to triumph in Christ, and maketh manifest the savour of his knowledge by us in every place."* [2]

Notice that scripture tells us "always," not just sometimes. Since death and life are in the power of the tongue, I began speaking victory "always" in every situation. There were times where I had much testing and sometimes long waits for results. Before I learned to call those things that be not as though they are, I would wait to see if the findings were good or bad with consuming dread.

What is the difference? I am no longer waiting in agony to hear if a report is good or bad. Instead of waiting as if the test result was my answer, I took the Word as my good report before the test results came back. Either way, if they were good or bad, I acted on the Word. I declared victory. I was and still am totally persuaded that His Word is Truth.

On my journey of restored health, I began speaking words that were powerful. I began speaking life, not death. What a difference that made in my life!

Truly, when we line up our words with God's Word, we can have what we say. *"Let the words of my mouth, and the meditation of my heart, be acceptable in thy sight, O Lord, my strength, and my redeemer."*[3]

WHAT IS COMING OUT OF MY MOUTH?

"For out of the abundance of the heart the mouth speaketh."[4]

I asked myself these questions: "What is coming out of my mouth in abundance? What is the dominant theme?" I began to reflect on the conversations I was entertaining with myself and with others.

Consider what you think about, because what you listen to, think and say in abundance will manifest or become evident in your life. You can pay close attention to what you think about and what you talk about.

I recall an old saying I used to repeat when I was a kid, "Sticks and stones may break my bones, but words will never hurt me." Interestingly, though, the words people say can hurt deeply.

Scripture says just the opposite, *"There is that speaketh like the piercings of a sword: but the tongue of the wise is health."*[5]

After my treatments were over, I returned home to live a somewhat normal life, or so I thought. A short time later, the doctor found other lumps, and once again the lion roared loudly.

Doubt, worry, and fear reared their ugly heads. The question jumped up, "Did it come back?" I recognized the wiles of the devil and refused to hold on to thoughts of fear. I decided to fight the good fight of faith again, and again, and again. It was a faith fight, not a fist fight—a fight to retain the truth of the Word in my life by casting my care and every thought at the foot of the Cross in total obedience of Christ.

Anyone who has gone through this journey may know of the many fears that lurk in your head concerning a cancer diagnosis. Do not succumb to the lies of the adversary. If the doctor says, "There is nothing more they can do," thank him, and be assured that with God all things are possible. He is the great physician in whom you can totally trust. Getting rid of every imagination and every high thought that is against the knowledge of God is the battle plan. The only alternative is to accept the devil's lies against the Word of God, thereby allowing him access into your life so he can he steal, kill, and destroy.

DECLARE THE VICTORY

Therefore, to experience victory in Christ, begin today to choose to form new habits of thought, confession, and action.

Overcoming deeply ingrained habits that have brought defeat in the past might take some hard work, but you can persevere with God's help and His Word. Trust Him and act on His Word. This is the step-by-step victory plan in Christ.

A new mindset based on God's Word is the key to power in life. Change your mind, change your life. My renewed mindset was, "I am not the sick pleading for healing, but I am the healed taking back what was stolen from me, my health. I am coming from victory, not seeking the victory. I already have the victory; the devil is a defeated foe, and I am strong in the Lord and in the power of His might. I am a commander, not a beggar."

I commanded those new lumps to, "go in the name of Jesus Christ," using the authority God gave me. After some difficult procedures, all was found negative and of no further concern. I have confidence and trust in God's Word, and I thank God for another victory. Now only life-filled words come out of my mouth. At times, fear jumps me, but I am assured from God's Word of His love for me. Because I know He cannot lie, I take back my position of triumph.

FIERY DARTS

Even during the writing of this book, there were plenty of fiery darts and obstacles thrown at me. I knew the adversary, the devil, would not lay out a red carpet for me to expose some of his wily ways and lies without a fight. I accidentally cut my eye and an infection developed. I was ministered to and was healed. The healing was progressive over a period of three weeks during the writing of this book. It took a good fight of faith to type several thousand words a week with one eye. I believed. I received both my healing and my completed manuscript.

In my life there are many obstacles or mountains to hinder my path as Mark 11:23-25 taught me. However, I have more understanding of the power I have to remove those mountains. The world may say, "Climb every mountain," but God showed me I can just remove the mountain. He also made it a point that I am to do it. I am not to wait for Him or anybody else to do it. He so lovingly gave each of us the power and authority to follow through with His instructions.

This book is written to anyone who has been robbed; in my case it was my health. What about mental health, spiritual health, and financial health? These are issues of life we can take back also.

This is just the beginning. Jesus Christ paid the price for our salvation and our healing. Yes, the price was paid in full. Therefore, it is the right thing to do. He gave us the authority. He gave us His name to use. So, take it back. Take whatever has been stolen from your life!

Recently, I had to have dental work that included having a partial plate made for a few of my front teeth. It was an uncomfortable situation. There was a rather unpleasant piece of plastic that fit in the roof of my mouth which I did not like at all. Then, shortly afterwards, I learned I needed three crowns on my upper teeth. This procedure had a rather large price tag along with it. I started to complain, and then an alternative plan was given to me. I could have all my upper teeth pulled and have an upper set of false teeth made. It would be less expensive. When I saw the false teeth, however, I immediately chose the crowns. Having a choice between the crowns or the false teeth was a no-brainer for me. I was now happy to pay the price for the crowns.

Life is a matter of perspective, how we look at things. Now, I have fully accepted my partial plate and the crowns were well received along with the price tag. In the same way, our health situation may tempt us to be unthankful, and to complain to God with comments like, "Why do I have to fight the good fight of faith with this disease, or this sickness, or this mental health issue?"

We don't have to fight. We have a choice. We can choose to not tolerate sickness and disease. We can choose life—we can choose to believe His Word that by His stripes we were healed. Yes, it may cost us something. It cost us labor to fight the good fight of faith, to believe we received our healing before we see it in manifestation or evidence.

The world seems to run on the premise of, "I will believe it when I see it." The Word of God works with the truth of "I believe it and then I see it."

THOUGHTS ARE SEEDS FOR OUR WORDS AND DEEDS

I would never invite a thief into my house. So, why would I allow thoughts that steal my joy to make themselves at home in my mind? I know my thoughts are important when I remember God's Word, *"For as he thinketh in his heart, so is he."* [6] My most dominant thoughts will become blueprints for my life's coming attractions. It is so revealing to consider what I thought about the most yesterday. If they were good, positive thoughts, I'm sure my day went well. However, if they were predominately negative thoughts, my day probably did not go well.

Thoughts are things. They have substance, and I am in control of what I think. I may not be able to control my circumstances, but I can control how I react to them. For example, my reaction to someone's anger toward me has the power to affect the condition of my health. At times, people might get very angry at you or me. When you hear someone's rants and harsh words and allow those words to penetrate your heart, you become sick inside.

I am learning to act on the Word of God that says to answer softly and diffuse that anger. One way that I can do this is to agree they might be right and then thank them. *"A soft answer turns away wrath."* [7] This usually diffuses that anger and keeps me in better health, both physically and mentally. And, perhaps the person may be right, but whether they are right or wrong is not where I put my concentration. I am in control by choosing my thoughts and my response. Those harsh words are not controlling me.

There are some scriptures that I began practicing, literally:

> *"Be careful for nothing; but in everything by prayer and supplication with thanksgiving let your requests be made known unto God. And the peace of God, which passeth all understanding, shall keep your hearts and minds through Christ Jesus."* [8]

When I depend on God's Word, I love the peace of God that follows. This has been a good schoolmaster ever since. I find myself going to God with all my requests for His help and guidance.

At my workplace one year, we had a manager who was well known for his bad temper and mistreatment of the employees. If anyone allowed his words to penetrate their heart, they would feel like a piece of mincemeat inside. My fellow workers would continually talk about him and curse him. He was a very angry man and could make our lives miserable.

My husband and I went to God about what I could do. He referred me to Luke 6:28: *"Bless them that curse you and pray for them which despitefully use you."*

I remember saying, "You have got to be kidding. This guy is a holy terror, and God wants me to pray for him?" That really was not what I had expected, but that was my answer from God, and I needed His power and help. I did it, day after day, and once again the Word of God was the solution.

One day, we all noticed this man was getting kinder. Eventually, he even began giving compliments. We were shocked and, wow, were we blessed. God's Word of instruction brought forth a miracle. I would never have thought to pray for the man or the problem. Again, I learned a valuable lesson.

So, when I say, "Thoughts are seeds for our words and deeds," I am so thankful to know His thoughts and ways. The thoughts of God that I decided to think, and the prayers I decided to speak for this man were the power of God's Words in action and brought about this miracle. (All I had to do was believe.)

This was another mountain that was removed.

"With God all things are possible."

Now, you move your mountains.

chapter 5
WOW, GOD, WOW

A scientist, Dr. Werner Gitt, published a study merging God's Word with scientific facts. The following data and information are from some of his writings in his article, "Counting the Stars." People have always been fascinated by the stars and many have tried to count them. When God promised Abraham that he would have innumerable descendants, He drew a striking comparison: *"'Look now towards heaven, and tell the stars, if thou be able to number them': and He said unto him, 'So shall thy seed be.'"* [1]

The total number of individual stars visible in both the northern and the southern celestial hemispheres is about 6,000. Thus, on a clear night one can see at the most 3,000 stars at the same time.[2] Is that all? With the advent of telescopes, many previously unknown stars were discovered. "Galileo (1564-1642,) using his homemade telescope, saw a ten-fold increase in the number of visible stars, up to 30,000."[3]

Today, the local "Milky Way galaxy, (of which our sun is a part), has been found to contain 200,000 million stars."[4] What an astounding result. "If somebody could count three stars per second, after 100 years he would have counted less than five percent of this number."[4]

Our galaxy comprises not only an unimaginable host of stars, but the size of this bright, starry band in the sky is also astounding. Its "diameter is said to be 100,000 light-years."[5]

"The total number of stars in the observable universe is estimated to be 10^{25}."[6] (That's the number "10" followed by 25 zeros!) In other words, no person knows the exact number.

What does the Bible say about the number of the stars?

Let us now try to visualize the above-mentioned number of stars, (i.e. 10^{25}). "No human being would live long enough to count such a huge number."[8] So, we will use a computer, one of the fastest ones available. It can do 10,000 million calculations in one second, which is blazing fast. Even at this great speed, "it would require 30 million years of non-stop counting to count the stars, but no computer could last as long as that."⁹ God has foretold the result of such an endeavor through His prophet Jeremiah. The stars are, to all intent and purposes, countless; just like the sand grains on the seashore.

Not only are God's thoughts higher than ours, they are also much faster. He actually can count the stars. God's thoughts and ways are far higher than ours. Not only can He count the stars, He has given each one a name, *"He telleth the number of the stars; He calleth them all by their names."* ¹⁰ The very next verse emphasizes His greatness: *"Great is our Lord, and of great power: His understanding is infinite."* ¹¹ And yet God is also concerned about each and every human being.

> *"When I consider thy heavens, the work of thy fingers, the moon and the stars, which thou hast ordained; What is man, that thou art mindful of him? and the son of man, that thou visitest him?' For, 'Thou hast made him a little lower than the angels, and hast crowned him with glory and honour. Thou madest him to have dominion over the works of thy hands; thou hast put all things under his feet."* ¹²

That is what God thinks of you and me. Wow, God, wow. He crowns us with glory and honors us. He has given us dominion over His works and puts all things under our feet. We have been given this authority. How wonderful is our Father! *"Is there anything too big for Him?"* I magnified and digested the scripture *"with God all things are possible."* ¹³

I spent time remembering the miracles in my life and in the lives of others. "Wow, God, Wow" is my daily focus on His greatness. I remember walking to school talking with God as if He were walking with me. I believe He was.

WITH GOD ALL THINGS ARE POSSIBLE

A road to recovery and avenue for healing for me was to keep my eyes on the many miracles I saw in my life and in the lives of others. I began a journal to record the miracles I saw and read about. I called it my "Book of Remembrances."

When I was sixteen years old, I was saved from a life-threatening rape attempt. It occurred the night before Thanksgiving. Women in our city were on their guard since six women had been raped and maimed that month. The rapist was still at large. My friends were careful to look after each other; we were mindful of the danger as the city was on edge. The mood in the city was tense, to say the least.

One night, I came home from a date about midnight. My mom and my aunt had just cleaned the kitchen table. Our table was just below the kitchen window, and I remember thinking how sparkling clean they left it. I especially remember thinking that Aunt Joe had never spent the night with us before. It would be the first and last time she would do it. She stayed in my bedroom, and we shared my bed. Thank God she did, because a little later after we both had fallen asleep, I woke to find a man crawling on top of me. I sat straight up, staring at a knife which he put to my throat. I could not speak when he said, "Lay back down or I will slit your throat." At that moment, my aunt sat up and began screaming. The man jumped off the bed and ran out of the house.

No one was physically harmed. I was able to describe him to the police artist, and he also had left his fingerprints on the kitchen table. He got in through the kitchen window that my mother and my Aunt had left so clean. We found out later that he was the one who had raped six other women in the city, and he had also used the same knife on them. That incident was a miracle to remember. God protected me, I was not physically harmed in any way.

That man was found after that night. It turned out he had been following me home from school, stalking me. He did not know that my God and I were walking together. He also did not know my aunt would be with me that one and only night of my life.

God is amazing! Keep Him close in your life. My "Book of Remembrances" keeps His miracle working power before my eyes.

I FORGOT GOD

Later in life, when I was twenty-four years old with three children, my husband and I lived in Berlin, Germany, just shortly after the Berlin wall was built. My military husband had been injured during his tour of duty. We were living in the American sector inside East Germany in the free sector of West Berlin. These were days of horror, with East Germans both jumping from the wall and being shot. Many escaped; many did not. My husband was sent to the free zone in Germany after being injured, and I was left in West Berlin with the children for three months.

Due to my husband's injuries, he was sent to Wiesbaden, a German town where he could receive care. I spent many a weekend going through "Check Point Charley" and traveling through East to West Germany on a slow-moving, clackity clack train as we called it. Afterwards he was sent to the States, and our family followed a few months later.

These were times of great tribulation in my life. I had separated myself from God and His fellowship. I had been more interested in my desires than His. I did not even pay attention to Him. My actions allowed darkness to enter my life.

My husband was sent to a town in Ohio for rehabilitation of his extensive injuries. I was sent far away to stay with my parents until living arrangements could be made for the children and me. A few months later we were assigned housing for military families.

After that began the endless days of driving to the hospital to visit my husband, always hoping that day would be the day the doctor would release him to come home. It would be eighteen months total before those words were spoken. I remember crying in the parking lot of the hospital after each visit; the situation seemed hopeless.

At times, I felt like I could not breathe. I had to blow in a paper bag to catch my breath. I even had thoughts I might be going crazy. I did not know anyone in the new area for a while, so it was lonely. Our children were one, two, and three years of age.

My grandma came to assist me, but it was too much for her. She suffered a heart attack while helping me. She did recover, but she had to go home after that event. One day our one-year- old, Kristin, somehow had gotten out of the front door and a neighbor saw her in the street. That day, I nearly had a heart attack. Life was difficult.

Eighteen months later, my husband came home. He looked like a war refugee, crippled, and very thin. He was going to be released from the military with an honorable medical discharge. Then what would we do? At that time no one wanted to hire a disabled veteran.

Finally, I remembered God. I remembered when we had walked hand in hand together in sweet fellowship. I remembered when He had talked with me and told me of His love in His Word, the Bible. I took out my Bible and began restoring my relationship with Him. I began seeking His guidance, His direction, His help.

Then, I met a very wonderful friend who was, to me, the sweetest angel this side of heaven. She took me under her spiritual wing and taught me of my Father's love again. I met her when God directed me to work for a certain cosmetic company. I sought someone nearby who could take me to the meetings. She lived in the next city but offered to take me to the meetings. During one meeting, a woman collapsed with an epileptic seizure. My friend immediately prayed for her, and the woman revived to a normal state of health. I was amazed to see this powerful manifestation.

After my friend drove in our driveway and parked the car, I asked her if she would pray for me. She did. She ministered healing to me, and the scoliosis that had curved my spine was gone. My back was straightened. She had not known of my spinal condition until she ministered to it and commanded it to straighten. I was in awe of the healing power of God flowing through her. God had given her a revelation and allowed her to minister healing to me. I was convinced from then on that is what I wanted to do: preach, teach, and heal in the name of Jesus Christ.

After those inspiring times listening to my friend speak of God's love for us, I began to fellowship with God again. It was a thrilling time for both my husband and me. We began studying God's precious Word. Our whole family went to Bible college for four years, and my husband was ordained. Last year, I was ordained as well. Now, in our senior years, we daily give our lives to answer His call into His majesty's service. We have served God for almost fifty years.

YOUR CALLING IS CALLING

I am so thankful for all that God has taught me. The refreshing truths that I continue to learn about the awesome power and authority He has given me to do His work. Thirteen years later, I am now living free from that dreaded disease, cancer. What then is my calling?

"For even hereunto were ye called: because Christ also suffered for us, leaving us an example, that ye should follow His steps." [14] After learning how to steal back my healing, I also saw in this verse that we are to follow in the footsteps of Jesus Christ. I know every journey begins with the first step, so I looked at some steps of Jesus Christ. I found some of these steps in John: 14:12-14:

> *"Verily, verily, I say unto you, 'He that believeth on me, the works that I do shall he do also; and greater works than these shall he do; because I go unto my*

> *Father. And whatsoever ye shall ask in my name, that will I do that the Father may be glorified in the Son. If ye shall ask anything in my name, I will do it.'"*

Further, reading in Mark 16:15 I found more steps or instructions such as:

> *"And He said unto them, 'Go ye into all the world and preach the gospel to every creature. [Notice preaching and teaching precedes healing.] He that believeth and is baptized shall be saved; but he that believeth not shall be damned. And these signs shall follow them that believe; In my name shall they cast out devils; they shall speak with new tongues ["If" is implied here]. They shall take up serpents; and if they drink any deadly thing, it shall not hurt them; they shall lay hands on the sick, and they shall recover.'"*

At the writing of this book, I am seventy-eight years of age, and God has given me the same opportunity that He gives anyone who believes Him. So, I am taking it. I see that He is an equal opportunity employer, and age is of no concern. He has a great benefit program also. I especially love His health insurance plan. Living in vibrant health every day is an awesome benefit. Imagine living healthy every day. What a truth. We are the healed, not the sick seeking, pleading, begging for our healing.

God has provided many avenues of healing for us to take to recover any health that has been stolen from us. Ministering gifts of healing is a work we are equipped to do. He has provided instruction for us in directives and get some on-the-job training. We are fully equipped to do the works. *"I therefore, the prisoner of the Lord, beseech you that ye walk worthy of the vocation, [calling], wherewith ye are called."* [5]— God tells us that we were called. We have a vocation, a life's work. We've got a job to do, the works of Jesus Christ, and He's equipped us for it. One of those works is to heal the sick, and they shall recover.

This calling is for all who are God's children. The question is, "Will we answer God's call?" In our present day, we are quick to answer our cell phone calls. We may even keep our phone at our side or even in our hand. We are ready to answer calls with enthusiasm and joy.

God is calling us to action. Our answer and response to God's Word is faith or believing. I asked myself, "Am I as excited to answer a call from God as I am from my friends on social media?" We have been individually and personally called to action. We can do the works of Jesus Christ. That is exciting!

USE YOUR AUTHORITY

"Verily, verily, I say unto you, 'He that believeth on me, the works that I do shall he do also; and greater works than these shall he

do; because I go unto my Father." [16] Therefore, the works that Jesus did are available for us to do. And, we put forth our faith or believing Him to do these works and even greater things than He did. He said that we can do them, and that means we have the authority also. It is absolutely amazing, the power we have been given.

I could see that Jesus Christ's works fall into three categories. "And Jesus went about all Galilee, *teaching* in their synagogues, and *preaching the gospel of the kingdom*, and *healing* all manner of sickness and all manner of disease among the people."[17]

Jesus taught, preached, and healed. He did not just provide instruction for information. This instruction is meant to be put into practice so that the learner or the hearer of the instruction can have something to start with. Jesus took the disciples teaching, preaching, and healing with all power and authority. They heard the instruction. He instructed them personally. He heard them preach; He was with them, so they could learn. They saw Jesus heal people. They had a lot of instruction in all three of these areas so they could put it into practice. They had on-the-job training.

Jesus preached or proclaimed openly. We might recognize this as a formal position that people held in the world—that of "heralder". This was more common in older times than it is today, but they practiced proclaiming openly. A proclamation was always given with a suggestion of gravity, formality, and authority which must be listened to and obeyed. It is not as simple as standing in front of a restaurant and encouraging people to come in. It was a very serious event usually ordered by the king. The person giving the proclamation expected the people to obey whatever he was saying. He had the authority of the king backing up his words.

Jesus healed all manner of sickness and disease as a service to people. Whatever disease or discomfort has been "eased", the service is the curing or restoring to health to relieve the disease. Those are the categories of the works that Jesus Christ did, which He wants us to do. And these works are not just a part-time job. It is more in the line of a business, employment, or profession, because there is labor involved in it—a lot of labor involved.

It is important to note that believing or faith is required in these works, and Jesus Christ promised us the ability and the authority to do the same works that He did. Jesus's disciples did not just sit in fellowship once a week. They got up and went out. They went out. They went forth. That is what God is calling us to do with our individual talents and abilities within our sphere of influence.

Now, all we need do is exercise our authority. We herald forth with expectation, or we command things to happen in the name of Jesus Christ. Require it. Demand it. We can minister to people and command that healing happens.

We've got the power to move mountains. Healing is God's greatest advertisement. Miracles draw people to Christ.

Take all that has been given us. We are rich beyond measure. *"Blessed be the God and Father of our Lord Jesus Christ, who hath blessed us with all spiritual blessings in heavenly places in Christ:"* [18]

Can you get any better than that? How much more is there than "all"? We are blessed with all spiritual blessings. And, the heavenly places are far above all principality, power, might, and dominion, and every name that is named—far above. It's far above cancer. It's far above colds. It's far above any name you can name. It's far above!

You may know that you are seated in the heavenlies with Christ and are looking down too. It is as simple as saying with your own words out loud, "Jesus is the Son of God," and believing in your heart that God raised Jesus from the dead. That's it. You are part of His body. Wherever He goes, you go. He is the head. You have all power; all might; all dominion. You have this same power that raised Jesus Christ from the dead. God's calling is calling. He does not cut us off, but the question is, "Are we answering the call?"

These are just some of the avenues of healing. The manifestation of the gifts of healing is the power of God in you which will defeat the works of the devil. We are commanders who command and enforce what is legally ours to give. The absence today of believing, miracles, and healing in the body or church has caused people to doubt the truth of God's Word. Many do not believe healing is possible. We can do the works of Jesus Christ, one of which is to heal the sick, and we have the authority. To quote my wonderful husband, "There's nothing to it, but to do it."

chapter 6
I DARE YOU

DARE TO DREAM

"*And the Lord answered me, and said, Write the vision, and make it plain upon tablets, that he may run that readeth it.*" [1] On my journey of living a healthy life with God, every year my husband and I inquire of Him, design a vision, and plan for the coming year. The plan includes our spiritual goals, as well as our goals and purposes for the next twelve months. I design a vision board with pictures, images, scriptures, and written goals that include plans to carry them out. I keep it where we can see it and envision ourselves doing and having these things in our daily lives. We have the results; every year, our dreams and visions come to pass. I am reminded of a quote that I love by Jesse Duplantis, "I've heard it said, 'The poorest person in the world is not the one without a nickel; it's the one without a dream.'" [2] Isn't that a wonderful quote?

Sitting in a rocking chair is not my vision of growing older. I see myself on daily adventures with God. My prayer to God is, "What can I do for you today?" That is part of my health plan. During these past thirteen years, I have vowed to live life to the fullest. I refuse to allow the thoughts and symptoms of old age or illness to remain. I have many opportunities to accept those symptoms; I just refuse them.

CAN YOU IMAGINE?

"And calleth those things which be not as though they were." [3] I began practicing calling myself healed every chance I got, no matter the reports. I began to imagine myself strong, heathy, vibrant, full of life, able to go and do. Then I began speaking those words out loud daily. "I call myself totally healed." If God's Word says it, I speak it out loud and bury it into my heart. I call this "voice-activating" the Word.

It is not enough to just say the words of the Word of God, but I must also believe it in my heart. *"For with the heart man believeth unto righteousness; and with the mouth confession is made unto salvation."* [4] Health and gifts of healings are all part of that salvation.

One thing that was important to my health was having a purpose, a goal, and a challenge. Many seniors lose purpose and feel unneeded. In the big body of Christ, we are all needed. How could we possibly get along without all our body parts? We could survive without some of them, but we would be impaired. There are some parts we cannot live without at all, like our heart. Once when I broke my toe, I not only couldn't walk for a while but until it healed, I was off balance. I really appreciate my big toe. We are all needed. "What would you have me do, God?" I asked.

"Trust in the Lord with all thine heart; and lean not unto thine own understanding. In all thy ways acknowledge Him, and He shall direct thy paths." [5] I obeyed. I trusted Him.

At age 76, I decided to finish college. I saw myself getting A's in all my classes, being on the Dean's list, and being invited into the National Honor Society, all before I began my first class. All these imaginations came to pass. Five scholarships and other awards for scholastic achievements and volunteer work came to pass as I had envisioned.

I have purpose. I have health. And, with God, all things are possible. If you can see yourself doing a thing, it is possible that you can have it and do it. God provided the best teachers for me. College tutors were amazing. And I am not finished yet.

We have a tsunami blessing from God in Ephesians 3:20. What you see and what you say are possible with God. How do

I imagine? Can I imagine being like a child at play? Children often say things like, "Pretend like you're a princess and I am the queen. I am beautiful, but you are wicked and ugly" etc. They literally see themselves doing what the princess does when dancing with the prince at a ball, for instance.

As in Ephesians 3:20, can you imagine the power of God working in you? If you can't see yourself doing something, you will not do it. But, if you can see yourself doing something, you can do it. Need a scripture and verse for that? Philippians 4:13: *"I can do all things through Christ which strengtheneth me."* In place of thinking about how you feel or focusing on what you see or don't see, call those things that be not as though they are, and see yourself healthy, vibrant, and whole, doing the impossible with God. If our goals are not impossible, they are not big enough.

What about the older you get, the healthier you get? That would be a tsunami blessing, would it not? Abraham and Sarah had to change their minds; at first, they believed it was impossible to have a child at ages 90 and 100 but they came to know that it was possible! I have another favorite quote that is from Jesse Duplantis, "Believe the unbelievable, receive the impossible."[6] It's doable. Today, and every day. I love thinking that way.

Do you know that God promised a long, satisfied life as a benefit of abiding in His shelter? He did in Psalm 91. And, in verse 16, He specified the word, "satisfied,"—not sickly, or boring, or lonely, but "satisfied." I am not satisfied yet because I seek to do more for and with Him. I dare to dream.

Many things that you may see today were unbelievable and seemed impossible or even crazy at one time, such as airplanes, cell phones, television, electricity, washing machines, light bulbs, cars, and on and on. If you can see it (imagine it), you can do it. *"Now unto Him that is able to do exceeding abundantly above all that we ask or think, according to the power that worketh in us."*[7] Imagine something; think it; then speak it in faith or with believing. God said in Genesis 1:3, *"Let there be light"* and there was light. We say, "Be healed," and the sick are healed. Step out of the traditions of religion into the sea of the impossible and unbelievable, because with God all things are possible. Journey where no person has gone before. You are a vessel of power, according to the power that works in you.

A great question to ask yourself is, "What is impossible for me to do right now?" Write down five things today that are impossible for you to do. Now, consider that with God all things are possible, therefore, doable. I remind myself that if they are not impossible, then they are not big enough. When I am excited and expecting them to come to pass, I am on fire on the inside. Life is electric with God.

Expect tsunami blessings every day. Expect those things to come to pass. You want to cause earthquakes in the enemy's realm which result in a tsunami blessing for you. Think it; say it; do it. God will do more than you think. God will do extra, but you cannot take it if you think it is unbelievable or not doable. You will ride on high places according to that power that work in and through you. Experience it. Become a testimony.

VISION AND DREAMS

God never just fills a cup, He runs it over.

> *"Give, and it shall be given unto you; good measure, pressed down, and shaken together, and running over, shall men give into your bosom. For with the same measure that ye mete withal it shall be measured to you again."* [8]

For the most part, the church has erroneously taught that anything above need is greed, but that is not the Word of God. The church preaches need, not desire, and, that is actually disobedience because God tells us it is better to obey than to sacrifice. *"Delight thyself also in the Lord; and He shall give thee the desires of thine heart. Commit thy way unto the Lord; trust also in Him; and He shall bring it to pass."* [9]

Where is your vision? Make your vision plain. *"Where there is no vision, the people perish,"* [10] or wander aimlessly. God has filled up your account, now withdraw what you need. Take it. God does not work in an empty mind. *"For as He thinketh in his heart, so is he."* [11] God does not work with an idle will either. We must be organized with a plan. "A dream without a plan is just a wish," is a wonderful quote from Katherine Paterson. [12] A great question to ask yourself is, "If I don't know where I am going, how will I know when I get there?" Keep your goal out of your reach, but never out of your sight.

FIGHT FOR YOUR DREAMS

While journeying through the process of maintaining my health, I was especially encouraged by God to have goals and dreams with purpose. I spent a great deal of time seeking His direction for my life and dreams. I love traveling, teaching the Bible, and oil painting bright, colorful landscapes, seascapes, and portraits. So in between all the medical treatments, procedures, and long travels from medical facilities requiring days away from family, I decided I would fight for my dreams. I already was fighting the good fight of faith for my health, so now I began fighting for my new, exciting goals and dreams also. I wanted to stay excited about them and to live them abundantly with great purpose.

Most every athlete trains with a good coach extensively for the race or fight, along with their vision to win. The best coach I know is God. During my time alone with Him, I began thinking, "What is it that really thrills my soul?" I asked God to provide His vision, direction, and knowledge to help me achieve spirit-led goals. He did. The main thing was to change my focus from the disease to my new, exciting dreams. Changing my focus changed my life.

Choosing to change your focus will also change your life. Do not focus on your feelings. Focus on your vision, your vibrant health, and the Word of God. Say out loud, "I am healed. I will live a long, satisfied life." Have laser focus.

Give yourself a target date and a plan of action to get there. Focus on being strong in the Lord, and in the power of His might.

Declare the victory to your opponent, thereby causing him to flee. Baseball pitchers intimidate and distract their opposition. Notice how they throw words of confidence and "chatter" at their opponent. They use bold statements like, "You're dead in the water, man. I got this game. I am the winner," all before they make their first pitch.

Declare yourself the winner before you activate your plan. "*I can do all things through Christ which strengtheneth me.*"[13] Fear is an opponent and fierce foe. Declare it "dead in the water" and declare yourself as the winner. Now, go on to win your dream.

One year, my husband and I made the decision to give all of our furniture away and put our remaining personal belongings into storage. We then moved to Portugal for six months. What an adventure! We were ages 73 and 76 at the time. We ran a Bible fellowship there and taught God's Word. We had many opportunities to minister healing and meet new friends. It was an adventure with God.

We had given all our furniture to our daughter and returned our leased car. We had been living in a rental home at that time, so we literally had nothing to return to. We were following God's lead and personally experienced the principle that where God leads, He also provides.

When we returned home, we rented our daughter's home; and, guess what—it was furnished with all our old furniture! How awesome is that? God provided. We obeyed the "Great Commission" and the authority to carry it out. All who are born again of God's spirit have this ability as well.

Our desire was to minister healing to the Portuguese people. When we minister, we impart to others gifts of healings. We can lay hands on the sick, and they shall recover. Certainly, prayer is tremendous, yet it is not the ministering of gifts of healing. God is the overall source of all healing. We have no power of our own, and yet, we minister His healing power to others by laying hands on them. God's power goes out of us and heals the sick. Just as the woman with the issue of blood touched the border of His garment, and Jesus said, *"virtue, [power], has gone out of me."* [14] That is the same healing power that you or I impart to the sick when we minister to them.

LIVE A LONG, SATISFIED LIFE

I discovered that it is God's will for us to live a satisfied life—a happy and long, satisfying life, one that you do not want to leave. I can continue to get smarter, and I do not have to expect to be old and sick. No—I say out loud, "By His stripes, I am healed." Thank God.

I struck gold when I found the 91st Psalm because it was the first time I learned of God's promise of protection and a long, satisfied life. I intend to live a long, satisfied life by doing these scriptures daily. *"He that dwelleth in the secret place of the most High shall abide under the shadow of the Almighty."* [15]

Where do you abide right now? Our abode is where we live and spend time for comfort and rest. It is usually a shelter from the elements: the sun, wind, rain, and threatening storms. It is a place where we can hang our hat and generally feel safe. Have you ever thought what it means to dwell in the secret place of the most High, and dwell under the shadow of the Almighty? You might want to contemplate what it would be like. It is God's offer of protection and hospitality, and a beautiful invitation to a personal relationship with Him—in other words, abiding in His shadow.

I heard this explained in this way: a hen in the barnyard has many chicks who play and scurry around the grounds. When danger comes, she does not chase after her chicks. Rather, she provides shelter by extending her wings as she calls her chicks to come and abide under her outstretched wings. The chicks who obey her calls run under her wings for protection, but the chicks who decide not to hearken to her calls will go unprotected. She will gather the chicks close by her side and then bring her wings down over them tightly, providing protection in a warm, safe environment. The mother hen does not chase after her chicks—she simply calls them.

In like manner, we who hearken unto God's Word and His voice, and abide in His Word, will dwell in safety. When danger comes, He calls us to the safety of His Word. He does not chase after us, just as the hen does not chase after her chicks.

We have free will to run to our Father's arms and abide under the shadow of His protection and warm hospitality. If we decide not to pay attention to God's call, we, by our choice, will remain unprotected also. We must make a conscious decision to dwell under the shelter within the shadow or protection of the Almighty. What a beautiful invitation—to be in a personal relationship with Him, abiding in His shadow.

I am learning a lot on this journey of stealing back my healing. While I was looking into Psalm 91, verse 16 stood out like a diamond to me: *"With long life will I satisfy him and shew him my salvation."* That tells me I could live a long life, and a satisfied one. I wondered, "What, then, is a long life, according to His Word?"

"And the Lord said, 'My spirit shall not always strive with man, for that he also is flesh: yet his days shall be an hundred and twenty years.'" [16] One hundred and twenty years is a long life.

All my life, I had heard life expectancy was around seventy or eighty years old, and possibly a few more years. That is a very common belief. Seeing that I had a choice in what to believe, I said to myself, "I have a choice, and I choose what God says over what the world tells us. I choose a long, satisfied life of one hundred and twenty years." This was a new and exciting change in thinking to adjust my core beliefs. Another thing I wondered was, "Is being sick with all kinds of ailments living satisfied?" No. "Is sitting in your rocking chair all day living satisfied?" Not to me. I refuse that thinking completely. I dare you and myself to believe for the long, satisfied life God promised in Genesis 6:3.

chapter 7

THE BEGINNING
OF THE BEGINNING

A NEW WOMAN

I began looking at women in the Bible who were dynamic, courageous, and committed, wonderful examples of women whose commitment to God brought deliverance to themselves and to others. There were days on this journey that fear and self-pity attempted to overcome me. I chose to no longer allow those feelings to dominate my thinking. I decided to run a mental movie of Ruth, one of my favorite women in the Bible. Why Ruth? She was in a difficult situation that was beyond her ability to handle. I was in a difficult situation beyond my ability to handle as well. Ruth's husband had died, leaving her in a very difficult position in her culture. She was a very young widow which was considered a curse. Her mother-in-law, Naomi, had lost her husband and both of her sons. Naomi had no other sons who could redeem Ruth and Orpah. Naomi wanted to return to her homeland and send her daughters-in-law to their mothers' homes. Orpah went home but Ruth refused to leave Naomi.

And Ruth said:

> *"Entreat me not to leave thee, or to return from following after thee: for whither thou goest, I will go; and where thou lodgest, I will lodge: thy people shall be my people, and thy God my God: Where thou diest, will I die, and there will I be buried: the Lord do so to me, and more also, if ought but death part thee and me."* [1]

I especially love Ruth. One meaning of her name is beauty. She was a beautiful woman committed to her mother-in-law, Naomi, and Naomi's God. The obstacles she faced were challenging, yet she chose to live victoriously. I related to her because I had decided in my heart to do this also. It isn't easy, yet it is simple. God honored Ruth's commitment and gave her favor as Boaz noticed and eventually married her. Ruth's firstborn son would stand in the ancestry of Mary and Joseph, the legal parents of Jesus Christ. Ruth was steadfast; she held firm to her convictions. I love that kind of commitment. Her

THE BEGINNING OF THE BEGINNING

life is a great example of a woman who fastened her mind on God's truth.

Every day is a gift, and I am so grateful to God for His lavish love. He gave His Son, Jesus Christ, so we could have eternal life. In my home town, I remember a huge billboard with the scripture in bold letters which read: *"For God so loved the world, that He gave His only begotten Son, that whosoever believeth in Him should not perish, but have everlasting life."* [2]

As a young girl, that word of God impressed on me to believe on His Son, Jesus Christ, and to have that everlasting life. I started my young life attending the churches near my home. My parents never went to church, but they wanted me to attend. That is where I learned about my Lord and Savior Jesus Christ, in whom I confessed with my mouth, and believed in my heart, that God had raised from the dead. Then, I had a new Lord. I was a new person. I had a new direction, and I had a new beginning with a loving God and my Lord and Savior, Jesus Christ. I was only eight years old, but even at that young age, I believed God had a plan for my life. Dreams of being a missionary in a foreign land burned in my heart. I wanted to be married to a missionary also. I remember telling my parents that I felt called of God to minister. That was 70 years ago. Looking back, God has never let me down. I did take God's Word to other nations. I did missionary work, and I did marry a missionary, just as I believed.

There was a period of time, however, when I was about seventeen years old that I let Him down. I no longer had a zeal for the things of God. I stopped allowing Jesus to be the Lord of my life and went full force into the ways of the world. The Word of God was no longer my guiding light. I wanted to do things my way until I had racked and ruined my life by my selfishness. Darkness came into my life, and all the while I still attended church doing my religious duty, I thought. It was thirteen years later that I realized my ways were not working. I began seeking the Lord again, seeking God's Word so that I could begin a new life. Even though I was saved, a daughter of God, born again of His Spirit, without His Word daily in my life, without His fellowship daily in my life, my life was full of darkness. I shared earlier how a very wonderful lady and friend brought the light back into my life.

I recognized the difference, and I did not like it. I made a 180-degree turn to return to His fellowship, His grace, His Word and His love. Then, my life radiated with His light once again. God *"magnified [His], word above all thy, [His] name."* [3] That is why I magnify His Word in this book and share the many scriptures that gave me my life and my health back. Without God's Word telling me *"I was healed"*, I would not have known how to take back my health.

It's the doing of God's Word that provides the results. And you are not waiting on God to do it—He's waiting on you to do it. He's waiting on you to resist the devil and use the authority He gave you, the power He gave you over sickness and disease. *"Behold, I give unto you power to tread on serpents and scorpions, and over all the power of the enemy: and nothing by any means shall hurt you."* [4]

"Power to tread on serpents and scorpions…nothing shall by any means hurt you." Nothing. You have been given His power, and you are sitting at the right hand of God with Jesus Christ. He's the head of the body, and you are a part of the body. You have got the power, and you have the authority. You submit yourself to God. You resist the devil. The enemy has no power over you. He must flee.

I like the example of the police officers that you may see standing in the middle of the street or at a traffic light. They stop traffic, and they let traffic go. They have the badge, hat and whatever they need to do the job. They might be small of stature or frame, with no real ability by their own strength to stop a car, but they have the authority. Their authority was given to them by the police department or government that sent them to do the job. In the same way, God has given you the authority in Him. You don't have it by yourself. He gave it to you, and to me. I choose to exercise it. How about you? We can do it.

NEWNESS OF MIND

My journey to health is on-going. I have heard if you always do what you have always done, you will always get what you have always gotten. I do not want to keep getting the same results. I am making many changes or adjustments to my daily habits to bring about a different result. This brings a newness of mind. In the Bible God calls it the *"renewing of your mind."* [5]

I became a new woman when I learned to renew my mind. It simply means to hold the Word of God in mind and act accordingly. The first verse in Romans 12 has the word, *"transform,"* which comes from the Greek word for transformed: *metamorphoo*. It is to get a new figure in mind. [6]

This especially appeals to me because I love butterflies. They go through that metamorphous in changing from a rather ugly larva to a beautiful, graceful butterfly. The larva can't rush the process or decide to stay in the cocoon to rest for another month or so. When the transformation is complete, its new life bursts forth as God planned.

My healing journey is exciting. It is putting this Word of God into practice and changing or renewing my mind. It takes some time, but I am endeavoring to continue that process every day to become what God says I am. I am healed because Jesus Christ paid for it.

THE BEGINNING OF THE BEGINNING

> *"I beseech you therefore, brethren, by the mercies of God, that ye present your bodies a living sacrifice, holy, acceptable unto God, which is your reasonable service. And be not conformed to this world: but be ye transformed by the renewing of your mind, that ye may prove what is that good, and acceptable, and perfect, will of God."* [7]

I am proving this Word of God in my life about health by changing my thoughts to agree with God's truth. Facts can change, but truth never changes. God cannot lie, and by His stripes I am healed.

To put God's Word in my mind and see it come to pass, I must do it. I must work at it. With the passing of each moment, there is a decision for me to make, whether I am going to act according to the world (walking by the senses) or be transformed by the Word of God. I choose to walk by the Word of God. I want God's results evident in my life. I desire to manifest the greatness of the power of God. I am changing.

This beautiful, graceful, butterfly process of transformation has a starting point. To renew your mind, you must start at the beginning, and that is to act on the scripture in Romans 10:9. You must confess (say out loud) the Lord, Jesus Christ, and believe that God raised Jesus from the dead. Now you are at the starting point for newness of mind. Then, keep going—put God's thoughts (His Word) into your mind. You will transform; you will change. That is how I learned to walk with the power of God and live it. I am loving it, and I want to share it with you! it is exciting, and I want to soar.

SOAR LIKE AN EAGLE

On life's journey, there are often situations in which our health or lives are threatened. Thankfully, the same scripture applies in every situation. God's got us covered. Once again, we must remember that we believe and call those things which are not as though they are, not doubting in our heart when we pray. We believe now, not later—not just when we see the victory, because we already have the victory in Christ. This faith or believing works for sickness, disease, mental, and financial problems. Pray, and right then believe you have it.

My husband and I were recently in a critical situation and needed an answer from God. It was not for healing, but for our safety. We experienced the threat of a hurricane approaching our town. This was a large category five hurricane. We are no strangers to these storms, but a category five storm was stronger than any ever to land near our home. We were encouraged to evacuate the area.

The storm was huge and anticipated to nearly cover our entire state. Where were we to go? We had to decide quickly. So, we went boldly to God and expected a prompt answer. God directed our steps to safety within minutes of our request. We

THE BEGINNING OF THE BEGINNING

traveled several hours away from our town to stay with an acquaintance who knew our situation and graciously invited us to his home.

"But they that wait upon the Lord shall renew their strength: they shall mount up with wings as eagles; they shall run, and not be weary; and they shall walk, and not faint." [8] We were soaring above the storm as we trusted our heavenly father to guide us to safety, literally.

Our expectations and needs were more than met. God provided an overflow. We had great rest, great food, and great fellowship with our new friends. We were doers of the Word and not hearers only.

At that moment when you are praying, believe you have what you are praying for. Receive it right then and you shall have what you prayed for before you see it come to pass. *"Now faith is the substance of things hoped for, the evidence of things not seen."* [9] We were protected and safe, resting in the center of God's will. Thank God, the center of His will is the safest place to be. We encouraged ourselves in His Word, standing on Psalm 91, the psalm of protection. We were abiding in the secret place of the most High, under the shadow of the Almighty.

Would you like to mount up with wings like eagles? Then wait or trust with strong expectation for the Lord and gain new strength. We can truly soar like eagles when going through life's storms.

> *"But they that wait on the Lord shall renew their strength, they shall mount up with wings as eagles; they shall run, and not be weary; and they shall walk, and not faint."* [10]

We lived that promise as we mounted up with wings as eagles. We ran but were not weary, and we walked but did not faint. Our strength came from Him, when we were so needy.

Eagles fly higher and faster than any birds in creation. They are about 30 to 45 inches in length, but their wingspan can be twice the size of the bird's length. Their wings measure over eight feet many times, which allows them to soar high in the heavens.

Eagles will fly into a storm when other birds fly away or hide from a storm. Let us run to God. Expect His guidance and protection from the storms of life. We had successfully mounted up on wings as eagles along my healing journey. Once again, we ran to Him, put our trust and obedience in His Word, as we soared safely above and away from the devastation of the hurricane.

There can be many storms in life. Yes, sickness and disease comprise many of them. But we can mount up on wings as eagles, as His promise says. Picture yourself above those storms as you take His promise to heart. Wait for the Lord with an intimate relationship of trust and obedience to Him.

THE BEGINNING OF THE BEGINNING

I stole back my healing, I tightly held onto it and when the next storm comes, I'll soar above it also.

Soaring never just happens. It is the result of work. We must win the battle, achieve newness of mind and take thoughts captive to God's Word. When you stand victorious, you can soar like an eagle above the storms of life which try to destroy you. Thirteen years after I stood my ground and took my healing back, my life is forever changed. At 78 years of age, I am soaring like an eagle above the storms of life with a renewed strength. It is my intent that anyone reading this book be encouraged. You, too, can take back what has been stolen from you—anything, especially your healing.

A NEW LIFE

As this book ends, new life begins. Every day is a fresh new day with new hope, new-found joys, as the mercies of God are *"new each morning."* [11] I am looking out my window, and I see the dawn of the new day breaking with bursts of blue and orange patches of sky, just like my life is breaking forth with bursts of new-found hope and love. God put color in everything, making everything beautiful for His children. It is hard to describe the sweet sounds of the birds singing. Who would have thought of that? Only God. I love those sounds. I can hear the ocean waves calming my heart in soothing pulsations while I write this morning. How sweet today's new beginning is—my fellowship with Him each day, and my thankfulness for His tender care.

My healing journey is full of light to guide my path. It is my heart's hope that you would find something from my life to be a strength and blessing to yours, my readers. I shared many scriptures in my story because they illustrate how wonderful life can be in His Word and His love as you and I endeavor to live by every Word out of the mouth of God. We can voice-activate a scripture and believe it, take it, and live it.

conclusion

Finally, the journey of "Stealing Your Healing" has ended. One can take many different journeys. I chose to take this journey with God to take back my healing. It was difficult at times, sometimes frightening and very exciting as well. The Word of God showed me the best journey to vibrant health for me. Thirteen years later, I continue to declare that, *"By His stripes I am healed."* The steps I took to victory are available for anyone who believes. Take His hand and His Word and take your first step toward your victory.

However, the thief continually steals from whoever allows him to do it. Just like the woman in Luke 8:43-48 with an issue of blood, I, too, stole my healing, as you may also. Our faith can make us whole.

I overcame the hindrances that were in the way of my healing. Forgiveness was an awesome key to deliverance because harboring any unforgiveness is a serious roadblock to receiving God's promises. I also found other keys to closing the door and locking out unbelief, such as knowing who I am in Christ; walking the resurrection walk of Ephesians; changing my thinking, and renewing my mind, to name a few. I am fully persuaded that what God has promised, He is also able to perform.

I continue learning how to move mountains; how to submit to God and resist the devil, and, how to labor to enter into His rest every day. *"Come unto me, all ye that labour and are heavy laden, and I will give you rest."*[1] I am laboring to achieve the ultimate peace and rest of the accomplished works of Jesus Christ. It takes determination and work, but I will rest in His arms of victory.

Life is an adventure, and with God, all things are possible. Believing for the impossible to come to pass is available. I do emphasize doing it with God, because without Him, I can do nothing. He has equipped me fully with His gift of His Holy Spirit. I have God in Christ in me, the power to heal the sick and raise the dead using His authority. Wow, God, Wow! You gave us the necessary power and authority. I declare in faith daily that because of what Jesus did for me at the cross, I am healed. What an awesome God. He gave His Son, Jesus

CONCLUSION

Christ, who gave His life so we could have both eternal life and healing.

I want to say, "Thank you, God; thank you, thank you, thank you!" The world offers other choices I could choose to live by. I choose to live by every Word of God, and I choose to glorify God.

The Beginning

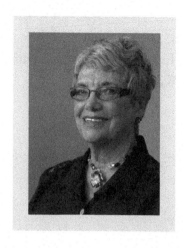

Shirley Ann Weidenhamer is a teacher, speaker, cancer survivor and victor. She inspires others to fight the good fight of faith and obtain victory over stolen health. Shirley attended additional college classes in 2017 and 2018 to challenge herself to learn more about writing and to further her education. She is currently writing about the "Adventures of Going to College in Your Seventies and Eighties."

Shirley has a drive to get fellow seniors moving towards their dream because it's never too late. Be on the lookout for her upcoming books on the topics, "Living Long and Strong," and "Daring to Dream." She and her cohort teach workshops on goal-setting and creating vision boards. For more information on these workshops, contact her via her Facebook page:

@ShirleyWeidenhamerInc

While they have lived in Portugal and Germany and traveled extensively, Shirley and her husband Ray currently live in Venice, Florida. Together, as ordained ministers, they travel and teach God's Word.

To contact the author:
www.WindowsOfHeaven.info

ENDNOTES

introduction

1. Ephesians 6:10
2. 1 Peter 2:24b

chapter 1

1 Peter 2:24
2. Isaiah 26:3
3. Psalm 107:20
4. 3 John 1:2
5. John 10:10
6. 1 Peter 5:8
7. 2 Corinthians 2:11
8. Mark 11:24
9. 2 Corinthians 2:14

chapter 2

1. Kenyon 110.
2. Kenyon 110.
3. Kenyon 110.
4. Psalm 107:20
5. Mark 11:23a
6. Mark 11:23b

7. Mark 11:24
8. Louw Vol. 4, 5.
9. Strong
10. Psalm 119:25
11. Psalm 119:159
12. Psalm 119:92
13. Proverbs 17:22a
14. James 1:21
15. Proverbs 4:20-23
16. Proverbs 4:24
17. 1 Peter 2:24b
18. Psalm 103:3
19. 1 Corinthians 10:16
20. 1 Corinthians 11:29
21. 1 Corinthians 11:30
22. Romans 10:10
23. Galatians 3:13
24. 1 Thessalonians 5:17
25. 1 Thessalonians 5:18
26. Proverbs 18:21
27. Romans 1:21
28. Proverbs 4:23
29. James 5:15
30. Romans 8:26b
31. Ephesians 3:20-21
32. Mark 16:15
33. Mark 16:18b

ENDNOTES

chapter 3

1. 1 Timothy 6:12
2. John 10:10
3. Ephesians 6:10-19
4. Job 3:25
5. Job 1:2-3
6. Job 1:1
7. Job 1:5b
8. Allen 34.
9. 1 Peter 5:7
10. Job 1:5b
11. Psalm 34:4
12. James 4:6
13. Proverbs 17:22a
14. Cousins pg. 43-44

chapter 4

1. Proverbs 18:21
2. 2 Corinthians 2:14
3. Psalm 19:14
4. Matthew 12:34b
5. Proverbs 12:18
6. Proverbs 23:7a
7. Proverbs 15:1a
8. Philippians 4:6-7
9. Matthew 19:26

chapter 5

1. Genesis 15:5
2. Gitt
3. Gitt
4. Gitt
5. Gitt
6. Gitt
7. Jeremiah 33:22
8. Gitt
9. Gitt
10. Psalm 147:4
11. Psalm 147:5
12. Psalm 8:3-6
13. Matthew 19:26
14. 1 Peter 2:21
15. Ephesians 4:1a
16. John 14:12
17. Matthew 4:23
18. Ephesians 1:3

chapter 6

1. Habakkuk 2:2
2. Duplantis, Jesse. *Everyday Visionary* pg. 39.
3. Romans 4:17b
4. Romans 10:10
5. Proverbs 3:5-6
6. Duplantis, Jesse. *Everyday Visionary* pg. 3.

ENDNOTES

7. Ephesians 3:20
8. Luke 6:38
9. Psalm 37:4-5
10. Proverb 29:18a
11. Proverbs 23:7a
12. https://www.azquotes.com/quote/860056. Accessed 12 December, 2018.
13. Philippians 4:13
14. Luke 8:46a
15. Psalm 91:1
16. Genesis 6:3

chapter 7

1. Ruth 1:16-17
2. John 3:16
3. Psalm 138:2b
4. Luke 10:19
5. Romans 12:2a
6. Louw
7. Romans 12:1-2
8. Isaiah 40:31
9. Hebrews 11:1
10. Isaiah 40:31
11. Lamentations 3:23

conclusion

1. Matthew 11:28

WORKS CITED

Allen, James. *As A Man Thinketh*. Winston-Salem NC: John F. Blair, Publisher, 2010 [1913].

Bible, The. King James Version. Nashville, TN. Thomas Nelson, Inc. 2003.

Cousins, Norman. *Anatomy of an Illness as perceived by the patient: Reflections on healing and regeneration*. New York: Norton (7th ed.), 1979.

Duplantis, Jesse. *Facebook, Jesse Duplantis Ministries* 29 November 2018: www.facebook.com/JesseDuplantisMinistries. Accessed 30 November, 2018. JDM.org.

Duplantis, Jesse. *The Everday Visionary, Focus Your Thoughts, Change Your Life*. New York, NY: Touchstone/Howard Books, A Div. of Simon & Schuster, Inc., July 2008.

Gitt, Dr. Werner. "Counting the Stars" Answers in Genesis. 1 March 1997. https://answersingenesis.org/astronomy/stars/counting-the-stars/. 27 February 2018.

Kenyon, E.W. *The Hidden Man*. Lynnwood, WA: Kenyon's Gospel Publishing Society, Inc., 1998.

Louw, J.P. & Nida, E.A. *Greek-English Lexicon of the New Testament: Based on semantic domains.* New York, NY, USA: United Bible Societies, 1988.

Paterson, Katherine. "AZQuotes.com, Wind and Fly LTD." *paterson-86-0-0-056.jpg* December 2018: accessed 12 December, 2018. https://www.azquotes.com/quote/860056.

Strong, James. *Strong's Exhaustive Concordance of the Bible, 7th Ed.* Abingdon Press, 1890.

All verses taken from the King James Version of the Bible.